Dr. Sebi Mucus Cleanse & Stop

7 Days to Cut Mucus Out Forever and Quit Smoking.

Meal Plan With 21 Tasty Plant-Based Alkaline Recipes Approved by Dr. Sebi

Kathryne Rose Miller

trademarks and brands within this book are for clarifying purposes only and are the owned by the owners themselves, not affiliated with this document.

Dedication

Alfredo Bowman was born and is lovingly known as Dr. Sebi. Thank you for sharing your African Bio Mineral Balance expertise and the strength of natural alkaline plant foods and herbs to reverse sickness and heal the body.

You became an information vehicle that changed our lives and made surviving for us so much simpler and more gratifying. In the face of challenges, we love you for the difficulties you have endured in sharing alkaline diet knowledge. Via us, you carry on. We will keep helping your legacy.

Table of contents

Introduction

Dr. Sebi is a naturalist, pathologist, biochemist, and herbalist. In Central and South America, North America, Africa, and the Caribbean, he has researched and directly experienced herbs and has established a unique approach and technique with herbs to cure the human body that is deeply rooted in more than 30 years of practice. The diet of Dr. Sebi is popular worldwide because of its alkaline, plant-based composition. When combined with unique nutrients offered on the diet's website, supporters say it decreases illness likelihood.

Dr. Sebi claimed that all the illness was induced by acidity and mucus. This diet stated that by alkalizing the blood, it would rejuvenate the cells by removing toxic material. He believed that the body should be detoxified by consuming some foods and eliminating others, creating an alkaline environment that might decrease illness incidence and symptoms. Western medicine to illness was considered to be unsuccessful by Dr. Sebi. He assumed that acidity and mucus induced all diseases, rather than viruses and bacteria, for instance. A central idea behind the diet is that only in acidic conditions will the disease survive. To avoid or eliminate sickness, the diet's purpose is to maintain an alkaline state in the body.

When we battle off an illness, often, the mucus becomes thicker. Because it can be slimy and runny as well, it depends on the kind of infection or irritant that stimulates the mucus-making tissues of the body. According to Dr. Sebi, if the mucus gets into the nostrils, the term for it is sinusitis. Name it bronchitis if the mucus passes down the bronchial drain. As mucus heads to the lungs. It's called pneumonia. And Prostatitis is whenever the mucus moves to the prostate gland. And they name it yeast infection n, vaginal discharge, or endometriosis as the mucus travels to the woman's uterus.

Therefore, for the Dr. Sebi diet, there seem to be eight main rules that should be practiced. Specifically, they rely on removing animal-related items and extremely-processed diets and would include proprietary body mucus expulsion supplements.

Sebi's nutritional guide has these rules that ought to be followed include:

- You are not allowed to drink Alcohol

- It would be best if you avoided Microwaves

- Canned and seedless fruits are not allowed

- Drink water daily (1 gallon of natural spring)

- Only restrictive foods are permitted, only from Sebi's Nutritional Guide

- Animal products are not allowed, like fish, dairy, and hybrid foods

- Products from Sebi's website should be consumed at least one hour before taking your pharmaceuticals

- You should also avoid wheat; you can only eat the natural-growing grains that are mentioned in Sebi's guide

On Dr. Sebi's diet, you have to eat certain foods and avoid these foods. Foods that are not incorporated in the Dr. Sebi nutritional guide are not allowed

- Eggs

- Vegetables or fruits (canned and seedless)

- Dairy

- Seedless fruit

- Soy products

- Red meat

- Poultry

- Fish

- Food from a restaurant, take out and processed food

- Foods with yeast or yeast

- Fortified foods

- Sugar, but the date and agave sugar is allowed

- Alcohol

- Wheat

- Foods made with baking powder

Dr. Sebi provides a complete guide on stopping your body from making mucus or expelling the excessive mucus. When combined, the nutritional guide with an added supplement from his website.

These are some factors that will contribute to the feeling of clogging, thick mucus:

- Excess of heating or air-conditioning, which may lead to the environment being very dry

- Not enough hydration or drinking enough fluids, and drinking fluids such as tea, alcohol, and coffee, this may dry up your body's fluid

- Very drying over-the-counter medications

- Smoking yourself or second-hand smoking

This is how too much mucus can damage your body by causing:

- Sinus headache

- Runny nose

- Cough

- Too much Sneezing

- Nasal congestion

- Sore throat

- Along with very, many serious diseases

Dr. Sebi also gives recommendations for those who smokes. By following these guidelines, you can take your lungs back to health, to the crucial purpose of extracting oxygen from the air and transmitting into your blood, and lungs also play an integral part in your body's health. Smoking harms your body by affecting these organs; specifically, furthermore, smoking increases the risk for lung cancer; it's also a risk factor for cancers of the:

- Colon/rectum

- Mouth

- Larynx (voice box)

- Esophagus (swallowing tube)

- Pharynx (throat)

- Cervix

- Stomach

- Myeloid leukemia

- Pancreas

- Kidney

- Bladder

- Liver

How smoking or second-hand smoking affects your body:

- Smoking increases the risk of the diseases, Chronic bronchitis and chronic obstructive pulmonary(COPD). Chronic bronchitis is a sort of COPD. The other type of COPD is Emphysema; this disease gradually terminates the person's ability to breathe. in the United States, Smoking is an inevitable cause of death

- Nearly one-third of coronary heart attack fatalities are attributed to secondhand smoke and smoking.

- Smoking is related to around 75 percent of cases of lung cancer.

- The number of people who smoke is still low, but too many teenagers still smoke, vaporize, and use other tobacco types, particularly between the years of 21 and 34 of age.

- About the kids, age 3-11 are prone to secondhand smoke.

- Smokers' life expectancy is less than10 years less than nonsmokers, on average.

- Although all hope is not lost, you can still start today and quit smoking, which produces excess mucus; the main cause of every disease. You can be one of the million people who stop every year and start their journey towards a healthy life by following Dr. Sebi's nutritional guide and tips and tricks.

Chapter 1: Dr. Sebi – How Mucus Works

Mucus, formed by several lining tissues in the human body, is a natural, stringy, and slippery fluid material. To prevent vital organs from drying out, it is important for body function and serves as a defensive and moisturizing surface. For irritants such as pollen, bacteria, and smoke, mucus often serves as a pit. To aid fend off pathogens, it includes bacteria-killing enzymes and antibodies.

A lot of mucus is formed by the body — around 1 - 1.5 liters every day. Until its output is enhanced or the mucus' consistency has modified, as may happen with numerous diseases and conditions, we do not seem to take notice of mucus at all. Mucus is composed primarily of water, allowing it its liquid form. However, there are also different salt and proteins in it. Specifically, glycoproteins that are sugar-containing proteins be called mucins, that give the gelatinous quality to the mucus. Discarded white blood cells battling infection plus other debris accumulated in the nasal passages sometimes take a ride in the mucus.

Mucus is a naturally protective fluid extracted from different body locations, such as the sinuses, mouth, intestines, stomach, and lungs. Mucus itself consists of various substances, but a substance named mucin is its main portion. Depending on their nature, the mucins in mucus can act as a lubricant, selective barrier, or viscous substance. Mucus covers surfaces all over our bodies. The structure and development of mucin are naturals, which lets us survive with several different bacteria. However, where the composition and structure of mucin are irregular, the disease may ensue. When you have an infection or a cold, and your nose flows like a water tap, you create an abundance of watery body fluids. At the other extreme, sticky mucus, generally the product of being overly dry, the sort that contributes to congestion, postnasal drip, and becomes crusty. Lung mucus is referred to as phlegm. Between our eyes or genital organs, it's thicker and stickier mucus. Such mucus is present in numerous ways, can be thicker or thinner depending upon the disease.

Allergens, bacteria, particles, and other debris bind to the mucus any time you take a breath and are then filtered out of the body. But occasionally, so much mucus, which involves regular throat clearing, may be created by your body.

Cause for excess development of mucus

There are a variety of medical problems which can cause the development of excess mucus, such as:

- Allergies, acid reflux, asthma

- Infections, like the common cold

- Several lung diseases, like pneumonia, (chronic obstructive pulmonary disease) COPD, chronic bronchitis, and cystic fibrosis,

Heavy production of mucus can result from different environmental factors, lifestyle such as:

- A very dry inside of the house

- Smoking

- Not enough hydrating the body, drinking fewer fluids

- Too much consumption of beverages that can make the body loses fluid, such as alcohol, coffee, and tea

- Drying medications

1.1 Diseases Caused by Mucus

Too much production of mucus can develop these disease's as well as many others

- **Asthma**

Asthma is characterized as a normal, chronic respiratory disorder induced by inflammation of the airways that causes trouble breathing. Symptoms of asthma are dry cough, chest tightness, wheezing, and breathlessness.

- **Chronic Obstructive Pulmonary Disease (COPD)**

The chronic pulmonary obstructive disorder is a collective word that includes many lung conditions that involve breathlessness or usual failure to exhale. People typically experience shortness of breath, sputum (lung mucus) typically coughs, particularly in the morning. For certain patients, COPD may be difficult to recognize, since signs are sometimes confused for the natural aging phase and weakening of the body.

- **Chronic Bronchitis**

A type of COPD illustrated by a persistent cough is known as chronic bronchitis. Particularly in the morning, people typically cough up mucus from their lungs). this is because of that in the airways. Mucus glands increase their production, and patients must cough out the excess secretion.

- **Emphysema**

An extreme respiratory disorder, which is another type of COPD, is known as emphysema. Smoking is the most popular source. Many that suffer from emphysema have difficulty with their lungs exhaling oxygen. The lungs' airways are impaired by tobacco smoke and mucus to the extent that they can no longer mend themselves.

- **Lung Cancer**

This cancer is hard to diagnose with the capacity to grow in every section of the lungs. Very commonly, cancer occurs around air sacs in the key part of the lungs. DNA defects in the lungs allow irregular cells to replicate and trigger unhealthy cells or tumors to develop out of reach. The normal activities of the lungs interact with these tumors.

- **Cystic Fibrosis/Bronchiectasis**

Cystic fibrosis (CF) is a hereditary (inherited) disorder that allows tissues, including the pancreas, the lungs, to build up moist, dense mucus. Thick mucus messes the airways of persons that have CF, which renders breathing impossible.

- **Pneumonia**

Pneumonia in the airways of the lungs is a chronic lung condition triggered by an infection. Infections can be infectious, fungal, or viral. Most individuals will heal within one to three weeks, but pneumonia may be very dangerous and often life-threatening for some individuals.

- **Pleural Effusion**

In what's considered the pleural area between the chest wall and the lung and is a collection of fluids, pleural effusion is considered. For a number of causes, like influenza, disease, or congestive heart failure, the fluid can accumulate. Patients typically recognize symptoms of growing chest pain and shortness of breath.

Many diseases are triggered by large quantities of mucus in the body that have been identified and researched, among many others.

1.2 Boost your Immune System to Fight Mucus

Here are a few suggestions to strengthen your immune system against the mucus

- Daily Fitness-Experts prescribe at least 150 minutes a week of regular workout.

- Eating a safe, nutritious diet: Dr. Sebi has a special diet rich in vegetables and fruits. Evaluate the portions and varieties of healthy foods that are the best for your wellbeing.

- Maintaining a healthier weight: Strive for a 25 and or lower BMI. With exercise and a safe, regular healthy diet, the safest way to lose weight

- Establish a plan and routine for sleep and exercise proper sleep health by having a better sleep.

- Including practices in your everyday life helps you relieve tension, such as digitally communicating with loved ones, getting outdoors, actively practicing yoga, running, creating art, or other hobbies. Minimizing stress and establishing healthy coping mechanisms.

- Quit Smoking-You will get therapy to help you stop if you are trying to quit smoking

- If at all, restrict the quantity of alcohol you hold in the house or reduce the number of bottles and glasses you consume, consume alcohol only in balance.

- Take precautions to stop infection-This entails regular cleaning of the hands and social distancing and paying attention to your diet.

- Take vitamins and other licensed Dr. Sebi herbs to battle body mucus, to live a healthier life free of mucus.

- Sometimes, in order to help the body function easier, individuals adopt healthier foods and food patterns coupled with exercising and continue in a recovery schedule., Treatments may range from medicines to oxygen therapy and cellular therapy. Always make sure to check in check if you or your loved one has emphysema, COPD, persistent bronchitis, or another chronic lung condition. Take measures to boost your immunity.

1.3 Foods That Boost the Immune System

Feeding certain foods to your body could help maintain your immune system healthy. These foods can protect the body from flu, colds, and other illnesses, visit the local grocery store can be the first phase. Design your meals to provide these strong food boosts for the immune system.

- Broccoli
- Citrus fruits
- Garlic
- Yogurt
- Ginger
- Spinach
- Red bell peppers
- Turmeric
- Papaya
- Green tea
- Almonds
- Kiwi
- Shellfish
- Poultry
- Sunflower seeds

The secret to healthy eating is variety. Eating only one of these things, even though you consume them constantly, won't be enough to help fend off the flu or other illnesses. Pay attention to the amount of portion and prescribed regular dose such that you do not get too much and too little of a specific vitamin. Eating well is a healthy start, and you should do other stuff to shield you and your health from the measles, cold, and other diseases.

Everyone is different, has various food sensitivities, has several dietary requirements, and is influenced differently by the foods consumed. For one individual, what works cannot function for another. With that in mind, when you attempt anything different, discuss adjustments to your diet with your dietitian. You should enjoy discovering the right anti-mucus diet for you in accordance with the above recommendations.

Chapter 2: Dr. Sebi- Mucus Cleanse

Mostly, whether you are allergic or intolerant to them, foods will trigger increased mucus development. Allergies may trigger more mucus production than usual in the body, and people dealing with chronic disorders may be more prone to experience allergies to some foods. Only a few suggestions and techniques apply to individuals when it comes to cleaning the body of excessive mucus. It is important to combat surplus mucus with a balanced diet and a safe lifestyle.

Everyone is different, and what makes mucus's development worse for one person does not make it worse for another. There are some items, though, that may increase the development and thickness of mucus. Usually, whether you are intolerant, allergic to certain foods, it can cause enhanced mucus development. Allergies may trigger more mucus than usual to be developed by the body. People dealing with chronic disorders may be more prone to experience allergies to some environments and foods.

2.1 Dr. Sebi's Mucus-Less Diet

The Dietary Advice from Dr. Sebi Diet provides us with instructions about what can be consumed in bulk and what items can be fully eliminated to cleanse the body from mucus. Here are mucus-thickening and mucus-causing foods you should try to eliminate from your diet with that idea in mind:

- Sweet desserts
- Red meat
- Cheese
- Butter
- Yogurt

- Ice Cream

- Milk

- Eggs

- Pasta

- Cereal

- Bread

- Corn and corn products

- Bananas

- Potatoes

- Soy products

- Shellfish

- Alcoholic beverages

- Candy

- Coffee

- Peanuts

- Cabbage

- Soda

- Eggs

- Soy

- Fish

- Milk

- Tree nuts

- Wheat

if your body creates too much mucus, continuously running nose, post-nasal discharge after eating, cystic white acne, and chronic eye or nose mucus, you ought to worry about what causes the response you feed, drink, or experience. It's the main allergenic diet for certain people: dairy, wheat, soy, eggs, tree nuts, and gluten. It may be an infectious disorder or a basic lack of zinc or healthy bacteria among some. Because the first stage is to figure out, eliminate the food that causes mucus, and, if possible, go on an anti-mucus diet. Unnecessary sugars and processed meats may also kill healthy bacteria and allow the body to develop mucus as a consequence. So whatever the condition may be, first find it out, and then incorporate some foods mentioned below.

Sebi Approved Dietary Guide Foods Naturally Containing Histamine. Your body produces histamine while you have an allergic reaction. Intriguingly, some foods produce some histamine naturally or help to enhance the development of histamine. Getting elevated amounts of histamine will result in more mucus being generated by your body. Chocolate, Bananas, strawberries, eggs, pineapple, and papaya can increase the amount of histamine. It is essential to bear in mind that certain foods can produce increased mucus for certain people and not for others. Before adjusting your food, please consult with your doctor.

Here is a concise overview of the ingredients suggested by the Dr. Sebi Dietary Guide:

- Vegetables like okra, Amaranth greens, wild arugula, avocado, turnip greens, bell peppers, chayote, onions, cucumber, tomatillo, garbanzo beans, watercress, kale, lettuce, except Iceberg, tomato; cherry & plum only, mushrooms, except shiitake, olives, dandelion greens, sea vegetables, squash, zucchini, and purslane.

- Fruits like Apples, pears, prickly pears, bananas, papayas, berries but no cranberries, cantaloupe, soft jelly coconuts, elderberries, oranges, tamarind, cherries, dates, seeded grapes, soursops, limes, figs, seeded melons, peaches, plums, prunes, seeded raisins, mango, and currants,

- Herbal teas(Natural)like fennel, Burdock, tila, elderberry, ginger, chamomile, and raspberry

- Grains like wild rice, Amaranth, spelt, fonio, rye, tef, kamut, and quinoa

- Nuts and seeds like raw sesame, Hemp seeds, brazil nuts, raw sesame seeds, "tahini" butter and walnuts,

- Oils like do not cook oil; Olive oil and coconut oil. avocado oil, grapeseed oil, hemp seed oil, and sesame oil

- Spices and seasonings like Basil, date sugar, bay leaf, pure agave syrup, cloves, dill, powdered, granulated seaweed, oregano, savory, pure sea salt, cayenne, sweet basil, tarragon, habanero, thyme, achiote, onion powder, and sage.

Teas

- Fennel, Raspberry, Elderberry, Burdock, Tila, Ginger, and Chamomile.

2.2 Herbs for Mucus Removal Dr. Sebi

Besides specify the food list, Dr. Sebi told about the beneficial herbs that naturally cleanse the body from mucus.

Seeds & Nuts which Include, Nut & Seed Butters, also

- Raw sesame "tahini" butter

- Brazil nuts

- Walnuts

- Raw sesame seeds

- Hemp seeds

Oils

- Hempseed oil

- Avocado oil

- Olive oil but do not cook it

- Grapeseed oil

- Sesame oil

- Coconut oil but do not cook it

Spices & Seasonings

- Herbs with Mild flavors, including thyme, basil, and oregano

- Spicy and Pungent flavors such as sage and onion powder

- Salty flavors like pure powdered, granulated seaweed and sea salt

- Tastes in Sweet like, including date sugar, pure agave syrup

Other Important Dr. Sebi's Diet Plan Rules

Additional guidelines to adopt, apart from keeping to the foods mentioned, include:

- Eluding all kind of animal products, which include fish and dairy, processed

- Avoid alcohol.

- Drinking as much freshwater as possible, daily

- eating Dr. Sebi's supplements and on a schedule

- Not letting the electric waves touching your food

- Not using seedless and canned fruits and vegetables

By incorporating these Dr. Sebi approved food lists, you can minimize the production of mucus in your body, which leads to the elimination of all the diseases caused by an excess of mucus

2.3 Food that Naturally Eliminate Mucus

Although it might appear that since many of the main food groups have already been filtered out, you should not consume anything, there are still several foods remaining that have the potential to minimize the development of mucus.

Cucumbers

Cucumbers are high in vitamin C, water, and potassium, which help cleanse the body. Vitamin C frequently enhances immune function. The alkaline quality of cucumbers often nourishes the intestine's lining and decreases inflammation of the digestive system, which also strengthens the immune system.

Ginger

Ginger Is a natural antihistamine and decongestant. By drying out excess mucus and stimulating the removal of its buildup, ginger's antiviral and antibacterial properties can help relieve congestion in the chest. Drinking ginger tea, a couple of times a day will help eliminate extra mucus.

Garlic

Garlic may be used as a natural expectorant and can aid in dissolving phlegm buildup. Garlic has anti-microbial properties, can help in combating bacterial, viral, and fungal infections, which causes respiratory glands to generate more phlegm. Having more garlic in the diet will aid in removing excess mucus from the body.

Broccoli

Filled with detoxification effects, broccoli produces enzymes that help to break down contaminants, and they are a good source of vitamin C. Their fiber often feeds healthy bacteria and help wastes escape the body ...hence no need to consume pills for detoxification

Carrots

Carrots can nourish us all on a deep level. Carrots are a gracious root vegetable that is so easy to overlook. Increased amounts of vitamin A, potassium that is the single biggest body cleanser, fiber, and high doses of vitamin c are contained in carrots, even farther supporting immune health.

Apples

Apple is such a star in easing mucus buildup in the body. Apples' vitamin C and fiber identified as pectin apples' potassium content contributes to their skills, and it is possible to enjoy apples in a number of ways. Eat them, mix them together, juice them up, or even bake with them. They will treat your immune system better.

Berries

Berries are yet another fruit well recognized for soothing the body, the vagus nervous system in particular, but that's not all! Berries are a great source of vitamin C, antioxidants, and potassium. They help detoxify the blood, and their fiber helps to minimize inflammation and infection by breaking down contaminants in the body.

Greens

Greens are among the most effective body-healing foods of all time; they sustain the body at every stage with healthy levels of vitamin B, A, and C, and potassium, also vitamin E. Cook at evening with greens, feed throughout the day or combine in the morning with them. Naturally, they purge the system of the body of mucus and contaminants, and their fiber may feed healthy bacteria, thus encouraging immunity and blood flow with its high chlorophyll content.

Oregano

With its high content of calcium, manganese, fiber, and iron, with a wide variety of other organic compounds, the nutrient-rich composition of oregano allows this effective herb an excellent choice for cleansing the body. Analysis has shown that by accelerating the toxin removal phase, oregano can improve liver function.

Tila Tea

Tila tea produces very helpful diaphoretic organic compounds, which indicates that they cause sweating, a very efficient method of extracting the body's contaminants, excess salts, bad fats, extra fluids, and foreign substances. For those suffering from fevers, Tila is often useful, since causing sweating can help lower a fever more rapidly and avoid irreversible harm to organ systems.

Burdock Tea

Bile development and digestive juices in the gut are activated by the same chemicals that give burdock its acidic flavor, making the liver absorb contaminants more efficiently and remove them from the environment. One of the liver's key functions is to remove contaminants from the blood, and burdock's organic components and compounds have been specifically related to enhancing this role.

Pumpkin seeds

A perfect source of omega-3 fatty acids that may help ease inflammation is pumpkin seeds. They provide magnesium, which decreases inflammation by allowing blood vessels to relax. Each of these nutrients will help minimize allergy-induced sinus swelling, allow improved drainage of mucus, and avoid congestion.

Chapter 3: 7-Days Program to Cleanse Mucus

This meal plan is designed according to Dr. Sebi's nutritional guide's approved food list. These meals will help you immensely in clearing mucus from your body. All these recipes are anti-inflammatory in nature, which indirectly causes no mucus.

3.1 1 Day Cleansing

Breakfast: Blood Orange, Carrot, and Ginger Smoothie

Lunch: Anti-inflammatory Lettuce Wraps(Vegan)

Snack: Any herbal tea from Dr. Sebi approved herbs

Dinner: Zucchini Noodles with Pesto

3.2 2 Day Cleansing

Breakfast: Apple, pineapple & spinach smoothie

Lunch: Kale Falafel Hummus Wraps

Snack: Garlic and Onion Sunflower Seed Crackers

Dinner: Cauliflower Rice Bowls **Turmeric, Ginger & Kale**

3.3 3 Day Cleansing

Breakfast: Green Shakshuka

Lunch: **Quinoa Stuffed Spaghetti Squash**

Dinner: Vegan whole-grain Ravioli with Artichokes & Olives

3.4 4 Day Cleansing

Breakfast: Spinach Artichoke Frittata

Lunch: Hummus & Greek Salad

Dinner: Garlic Miso and Onion Soup

3.5 5 Day Cleansing

Breakfast: Turmeric, apple smoothie

Lunch: Cardamom Coconut Chia Pudding

Snack: Any herbal tea from Dr. Sebi approved herbs

Dinner: One-pot Zucchini Mushroom Pasta

3.6 6 Day Cleansing

Breakfast: Strawberry & Spinach Super Smoothie

Lunch: Onion Soup with Apple

Snack: Anti-Inflammatory, Bliss Balls

Dinner: Arugula and Strawberry Salad with Cayenne Lemon Vinaigrette

3.7 7 Day Cleansing

Breakfast: Turmeric smoothie

Lunch: Kale & Golden Beet Salad

Snack: Any herbal tea from Dr. Sebi approved herbs

Dinner: **Savory Avocado Wraps**

All these recipes are rich in nutrients that, with the aid of Dr. Sebi's official nutritional guide, enable the body to get rid of mucus and inflammation naturally. You can also drink more water, use allowed herbal teas, increase the usage of ginger, cayenne pepper, garlic, black pepper, pumpkin seeds, oregano, broccoli, apples and pineapples, vinegar, dried fruits, avocados, tomatoes, spinach, mushrooms, eggplants.

Chapter 4: The Link between Mucus & Smoke

One of the greatest dangers confronting humanity today is smoke. Four million people are killed per year from smoking, and the figure is projected to increase to 10 million per year deaths in 2020. Tobacco use induces extreme addiction; about 85-90 percent of one hundred people who use tobacco would become addicted.

For tobacco consumers, nicotine in tobacco is the primary source of this addiction. According to an analysis carried out by researchers, tobacco smoking has been associated with overproduction of mucus correlated with recurrent bronchitis. The research shows that tobacco smoke suppresses an enzyme that induces mucus-producing cells to die spontaneously in the airways of patients with bronchitis. Previous findings have shown that the overproduction of mucus cells is prevalent in tobacco users' broad and narrow airways. Such overproduction is liable for airway congestion and diminished lung capacity in the narrow airways and chronic COPD's pathogenesis in bad situations.

Chronic mucus hypersecretion (CMH) is prevalent in smokers and is linked with regular obstructive pulmonary disease production and progression. Previous experiments indicate that up to 30 percent of the airway lining cells experience death after inflammatory reactions and revert to their original cell numbers. Also, this cell death is assisted by proteins. Disruption of this regeneration mechanism will lead to a permanent rise in the number of mucus cells and contribute to narrowing the airway seen in chronic lung diseases like chronic bronchitis.

In order to recognize smoke affects your sinuses, you need to learn about your nose and sinuses that they help maintain you safe. In your sinuses, nose, and the membranes are continuously developing mucus that serves as a defensive shield for the whole respiratory system. The lining of the lungs is the same as the lining of the nose and sinuses. There are many cilia or small hair-like structures that filter mucus, airborne particulate matter, and bacteria from the lungs, nose, and sinuses. Smoking allows the cilia, which naturally leads the user to elevated lung and sinus infections, to stop functioning.

According to research, all the mucus moves to the back of your throat where you ingest it, the sinuses and nose create between one or two quarts of mucus each day. The mucus starts accumulating in the sinuses, as the cilia are damaged by smoking and bacteria tend to grow there. A sinus infection may contribute to this. It begins to irritate the whole upper airway as long as you inhale cigarette smoke. Unpleasant gases such as formaldehyde and ammonia cause more mucus to be formed in your nose and sinuses.

4.1 In Ways Smoking Affects Your Sinuses

- The nasal passages' lining is affected by smoke.

- There are hair-like cells called cilia filling the nasal passages, which travel back and forth. By attracting infected spores, they operate with mucus to avoid contamination and then "sweeping" them free, expelling the possible infection out of the body.

- The substances found in nicotine are harmful to cilia and hinder function, such as ammonia hydrogen cyanide. Without activity, the nasal passages have an accumulation of mucus.

- The likelihood of infection is raised by smoking.

- The sinuses are the first defensive line of the body against foreign objects. The cilia and mucus in the nasal passages will do their work when subjected to irritants such as pollen or mild smoke levels and clear the selections quickly. However, large smoke concentrations will hinder the body's capacity to brush away dangerous bacteria and viruses, effectively opening the body's doors to pathogens.

- Linked to a compromised immune system, smokers tend to become ill more frequently and more quickly than non-smokers. Many young smokers are at great risk for contracting pneumonia despite being reasonably well.

- Smokers endure persistent face discomfort and headaches.

- Facial discomfort is widespread in smokers as a sign of persistent sinusitis. Nasal passages can become obscured without the activity of the cilia. This triggers irritation and pain from the cheekbones to the bridge of the nose to under the eyes. In the above back teeth, which are near the sinuses, the discomfort can manifest as strain.

- It is impossible for smokers to sleep throughout the night.

- In the pathways that contribute to the lungs, the paralyzing impact of tobacco smoke on nasal cilia often controls the cilia. People who smoke can feel congested without the cilia moving together with irritants and wake up coughing because of mucus's accumulation.

- There is also a possibility that smokers could experience sleep apnea. Smokers are 2.5 significantly more likely to have sleep apnea, according to a report, since tobacco smoking triggers swelling that limits air movement.

Smoking may be linked to a variety of other respiratory concerns such as:

- Persistent coughing & mucus

- long-lasting nose allergy

- Bad breath and bad taste of the mouth and

- Diseases of gum and teeth

- Weakened throat and mouth membranes, and amplified bleeding of gums

- Higher chance of continuous upper airway inflammation such as the throat and pharynx

- Throat and mouth cancer

- Vocal cords and pharynx cancer

4.2 Benefits of Quitting Smoke

Here are some benefits to quit smoking

- In the Brain, the cycle of addiction is broken, quit smoking will refresh the Brain and eventually break the addiction cycle. The vast amount of nicotine receptors in the brain will adjust to regular amounts after around a month of quitting

- Hearing becomes sharp, quit smoking will hold the hearing clear. even slight hearing loss can trigger issues like not recognizing instructions correctly and performing a job wrong

- Better Visibility, if you stop smoking, it will boost your night vision and help protect your vision by avoiding the harm that smoking brings to the eyes.

- Clean Mouth, yellow teeth and bad breath are not something attractive. After just a few days without smoke, the face would be brighter. Not smoking will indeed keep the mouth safe for the coming years.

- Brighter skin, quitting cigarettes is stronger than anti-aging lotion. Quitting may help cover up blemishes and prevent the skin from premature aging and wrinkling.

- Heart risks minimized, the main cause of cardiac problems and heart failure is smoke. Yet by actually stopping smoke, all of these heart problems may be eliminated. Quitting will almost instantly increase the blood pressure and heart rate. Within a day, the chance of a heart attack decreases.

- No Blood clots, another result of stopping smoking is that the blood may become healthier and less prone to develop harmful blood clots. Your heart would now have less job to do, so it would be forced to pump the blood across the body more quickly.

- Low level of Cholesterol, quitting smoking cannot get rid of the fatty deposits that are still present. However, it will reduce the cholesterol and oils present in your blood, which can help prevent the formation of fresh fatty deposits in the arteries.

- Cilia's Return, once you stop smoking, Cilia starts to regrow and restore natural function very rapidly. These are one of the first curing items in your body. When they first stop smoking, people often find they cough more than normal. This is an indicator that the cilia are returning to life. So while you're dealing well with cilia, you're quite likely to fend off colds and illnesses.

- Chance of cancer becomes Low, giving up smoking can avoid the incidence of new DNA harm and help fix the damage already done. The easiest approach to reduce the chances of developing cancer is to stop smoking quickly. Quitting smoke reduces the risk of kidney cancer, lung cancer, bladder cancer, pancreatic cancer and esophageal cancer

- Belly fat is gone, quitting smoking can decrease your body fat and reduce your chance of getting diabetes. If you have diabetes now, stopping will help you maintain your blood sugar levels under control.

- Standard Amounts of Estrogen, if a woman once stops smoking, the hormone levels will slowly return to usual. And if you're planning to have kids eventually, quitting smoking right away can improve the potential odds of a successful pregnancy.

- Avoid lung tissue damage, scarring of the lungs is not temporary. That is why it is necessary to stop smoking before you do irreversible harm to your lungs. After two weeks after leaving, you may find it's easier to walk up the stairs, and you might be less out of breath. Don't delay until later; leave the cigarettes now.

- Prevent Emphysema, there is no treatment for emphysema. Although stop smoking when you are young until you have done years of harm to the fragile air sacs in the lungs, it will better prevent you from developing emphysema after years to come.

The Immune System and Blood

- Standard Count of White Blood Cells, your body will continue to recover from the accidents sustained by smoking after you stop smoking. White blood cell levels finally return to usual and are no longer on the defensive.

- Effective Healing, Blood supply to wounds can be increased by avoiding smoking, enabling vital nutrients, vitamins, and oxygen to enter the wound to recover better.

- Immune System Strength, your nervous system is no longer susceptible to tar and tobacco after you start smoking. It's going to get better because you're going to become less likely to get ill.

- Bones and Muscles become strong.

- Giving up smoking will greatly boost your blood oxygen availability, and muscles will become healthier and stronger

- Stronger Bones, stopping smoking can, now and in later life, lower your risk of fractures. make your bones start now

- Smokers have an increased risk of depression and anxiety, though the reason for this is unclear. To feel healthier, you could vape. You may feel more stressed and sad when you stop smoking. Insomnia is still widespread, too. A severe problem is a depression. It's better to handle it with a specialist who may prescribe conversation therapy, drugs, or light therapy

Chapter 5: Quit Smoking with Dr. Sebi

Lungs keep the human body Alkaline, and assist in the body's pH equilibrium. They raise the rate of breathing to remove carbon dioxide faster as they sense a spike in acidity. They filter Blood Clots. The lungs flush away tiny blood clots from the bloodstream to escape 'fluid embolisms.' They safeguard the heart. In some kinds of crashes, the lungs act as a kind of airbag for the heart, sustaining the impact and shielding it. They safeguard your body against infection. The lungs trap pathogenic agents that trigger inflammation and, by exhalation, remove them from the body.

They regulate blood supply. At any time, the lungs will adjust how much blood they hold. For example, during exercise, as they engage with the heart to make it perform more effectively, this role may be beneficial. They help detox your body. Seventy percent of pollution is removed from the lungs only by simply breathing.

5.1 Dr. Sebi's Tips to Stop Smoking

- Avoid smoking. If you're Dr. Sebi's nutritional guide follower, so you realize that smoking is a big NO. The air openings in the lungs are restricted by tobacco smoke, and it makes breathing more challenging. It induces lung swelling or persistent inflammation, which may contribute to recurrent bronchitis. Lung cancer and persistent obstructive pulmonary disorder (COPD) are among the primary factors, not to mention numerous other diseases, such as cardiac failure, high blood pressure, asthma, erectile dysfunction, loss of vision, rheumatoid arthritis, and bladder cancer. To preserve your immune tract and protect your lungs, it is never too late to stop smoking. Dr. Sebi's will help you battle the cravings when cleaning the body at a molecular level if you're attempting to leave.

- Stop second-hand smoke. Passive smoking may be as dangerous as firing up your cigarette smoke. Secondhand smoking triggers 42,000 fatalities from heart failure and 3,400 losses from lung cancer each year. It's also not going to cut open a window or power off a fan, make sure you make your vehicle and home are free of smoke, and remind people near you not to smoke to preserve your respiratory system.

- Stop particle emissions from outside. Contaminated air accelerates the lungs' aging and raises the likelihood of chronic lung disease. It even leaves the lungs, nasal passages, and throat sore. Start monitoring the air quality levels in your region to safeguard yourself, take care of your health, and stop going outdoors while they are contaminated air. Cough / Cold Herbal Tea from Dr. Sebi can help you ease the symptom's link with outdoor air pollution. A device that can screen away up to 95 percent of the chemicals and small particles that make up air pollutants may also be used. Filling your house or workplace with indoor plants is another thing you should do. Plants will help keep toxins away and disinfect the environment surrounding you and your loved ones while enhancing well-being and healing.

- Must eat healthy and balanced food. Sticking to the Dietary Guide from Dr. Sebi will help maintain safe lungs and improve the immune system to combat infections. As dry lungs are more vulnerable to inflammation, water is also important for good lungs, keeping the required gallon of spring water drinking every day.

- The workout. Having enough exercise allows your lungs healthier and effective at supplying the oxygen that your body requires. It also helps to improve the potential of the body to combat germs that might cause you ill. The Immune Protection Herbal Tea from Dr. Sebi often helps preserve the lungs and immune system's health. Elderberries, the key component, lowers swelling and relieves nasal inflammation in the mucous membranes, like the sinuses. It's great for improving the immune system and taking control of the lungs.

Quick Advice

Decide to stop smoking completely and happily, work hard to prevent depressive feelings.

Make a list of all the factors that you would like to avoid smoking.

Start physically preparing yourself by consistently exercising, consuming lots of water, receiving enough sleep, and lowering your stress levels in life.

5.2 10 Herbs to Quit Smoking

- **Combination of Peppermint, Echinacea, and Sage**

Sore Throat Spray of Echinaforce can help you clear things up. If your throat is quite sore. Peppermint, Echinacea, and sage work easily to soothe and freshen your sore throats in this unusual blend.

- **Ivy & Thyme**

Thin phlegm can be improved by a tincture containing ivy and Thyme to promote chest expansion and alleviate bronchial spasms. In order to dislodge secretions, these plants function quickly. If you are too much coughing, you're able to cough less because your cough will be a good one when you do. In the battle against chest inflammation, Thyme is very strong. It creates high essential antiseptic oils that are categorized as naturally anti-fungal. and antibiotic Thyme is popular for a natural treatment that is cheaper than pricey drug creams, gels, and lotions to make things better

Thyme tea has the ability to evade away microbes and viruses and kill them, so it may function if the illness is focused on one. Thyme has been in use since ancient times as a lung treatment and is commonly used today to avoid and cure diseases of the respiratory tract and bacterial pneumonia.

- **Essential Oils to Inhale**

Through inhaling steam created from finely salted water and essential oils of plants like rosemary and eucalyptus, you can maintain the mucus membranes moist. Some drops of these essential oils can even be applied on a towel, and you should inhale deeply to clear the nasal passages. Any essential oils in the chest will alleviate breathing and remove the mucus. Some can also avoid bacteria known to infect the respiratory tract from growing.

Beneficial essential oils that will help you include:

- Lemongrass
- Basil
- Eucalyptus
- Peppermint
- Rosemary
- Thyme
- Cinnamon bark
- Tea tree
- Oregano
- **Spruce Buds**

Spruce bud extract might do a lot of good if you have a chronic cough. Santasapina Calming Syrup, suggested for the treatment of symptoms linked with mucus secretions in the airways, tends to remove contaminants that can block the lungs, due in no small part to the antibacterial and antiseptic qualities of spruce buds.

In addition to diluting secretions for almost two hours, the natural sugars have promoted chest expansion, but often give it a good taste.

- **Licorice Root**

On the globe, licorice is one of the most commonly eaten herbs. It appears in more recipes than just about any other single herb in Classical Chinese Medicine, and it is believed to harmonize the function of all other herbs.

Licorice softens and is calming for the throat's mucous membranes and, in particular, the stomach and the lungs, thereby cleaning every inflamed mucous membrane that requires help from the immune system.

- **Coltsfoot**

For hundreds of years, Coltsfoot has been historically used by Native Americans to protect the lungs. Large amounts of mucus from the bronchial tubes and lungs and were cleared out.

- **Osha root**

Osha is that herb specific to the Rocky Mountain region, which has traditionally been used for Native Americans' pulmonary help. The roots of plants include other compounds and camphor that make it one of the strongest therapeutic herbs for lung help in the world. One of Osha root's key advantages is that it improves airflow to the lungs, making it possible to breathe deeply. Also, Osha root is not an actual antihistamine, causing a similar impact when seasonal allergies flare up the sinuses and help relax respiratory irritation.

- **Oregano**

While oregano contains the nutrients and vitamins needed by the immune system, rosmarinic acid and carvacrol are its key advantages. Natural medicines such as oregano include substances that function as natural decongestants and reducers of histamine that specifically support the respiratory tract and the nasal airway's ventilation. Oregano oil protects from Staphylococcus aureus, a deadly bacterium, stronger than the other effective antibiotic therapies. Oregano provides so many medicinal advantages that everyone's medication cabinet could include a bottle of herbal oregano oil.

- **Lobelia**

According to a study, the lobelia-treated horses are able to breathe more easily. Its advantages are not confined to passengers. Appalachian traditional medicine was used as an 'asthmador.' Lobelia is considered one of the most important natural medicines in nature by some sources. Lobelia inflata extracts include lobelin, which has demonstrated promising benefits in the therapy of multidrug-resistant tumor cells. Lobelia produces an alkaloid known as lobeline, which breaks up friction by thinning mucus.

Besides, Lobelia triggers epinephrine secretion in the adrenal glands, which relaxes the airways and makes it easier to breathe. Also, it is included in many cough and cold remedies because Lobelia helps to relax smooth muscles. Lobelia should be part of the respiratory assistance regimen for all of us.

- **Elecampane**

For several years, Native Americans have used Elecampane to resolve excess mucus that influences lung function. It is recognized as a natural lung antibacterial agent, helping reduce infection, especially for individuals prone to lung infections such as bronchitis.

5.3 Food List to Reverse Smoking Now

Whether you smoke and wish to avoid and quit smoking, so there all hope is not lost. By consuming more of these ingredients, you can reduce the urge to smoke. They help combat nicotine addiction, which leads to reversing the signs and finally stopping smoking.

Fruits & Vegetables

Cigarettes prevent essential nutrients, such as vitamins C, calcium, and vitamin D, from being absorbed. Smoking only one cigarette, for example, removes 25 mg of vitamin C from the body. As some evidence indicates, these nutrients can be recovered by adding more vegetables and fruits into your diet, which can help minimize nicotine cravings. Food begins to taste good, and tastes are more evident after you decide to avoid smoking. You can also appreciate these foods more.

Ginseng tea

Any evidence indicates that ginseng may be beneficial for nicotine addiction since the role of dopamine in the brain, a pleasure-associated neurotransmitter, that is activated while smoking cigarettes, could be diminished. Drinking ginseng tea may reduce smoking's charm and render it less fun.

Dairy & Milk

Smokers claimed that consuming milk made cigarettes taste poor; most smokers said it added a bitter, foul taste to cigarettes. Drinking milk and other dairy items that make cigarettes taste foul may help discourage cigarette smokers when confronted with a craving.

Sugar Free Gum & Mints

When smokers get an impulse to smoke, chewing gum and mint will keep your mouth full. Moreover, all gum and mint work for a long time, generally more than smoking a cigarette. It would help to recognize what to avoid eating while attempting to quit smoking, too. some foods like meat, spicy foods, sugar, alcohol, and caffeine trigger craving for cigarettes and smoke, and elevate the taste of smoking

Although consuming and drinking the right foods will make it easier to avoid the smoke, it will increase the odds of completion and leave for good. popcorn, Frozen seeded grapes, cinnamon, crunchy vegetables, peanuts, and beans

Honey & Ginger

Ginger has strong medicinal effects; that is why the cure for colds is also ginger. Ginger, though doing well to dislodge persistent mucus, helps soothe the airways and ease coughs. Honey has antifungal, antibacterial effects, ideal if your airways are clogged with phlegm, and you have a sore throat or cough. Honey puts on the throat a defensive coating, reducing inflammation and helping the mucous membranes to recover.

To use honey and ginger effectively. Warm two tablespoon of honey, but do not let the temperature be higher than 40C, because honey loses its effectiveness on above 40 C mix with one teaspoon of grated ginger. Eat it for persistent cough for two-three days.

Turmeric

Turmeric is a veritable super-food. It eases discomfort, lowers stress, and improves the body's resilience, exactly as the doctor says. In, a glass of hot non-dairy milk, mix turmeric and black pepper, half a teaspoon each of, add a tiny spoonful of honey. This delicious concoction should be drinking regularly until the mucus clears away.

Any research shows that respiratory viruses that could be accountable for excess mucus, by eating these foods, it may ease the mucus and symptoms:

- Pomegranate
- Berries
- Guava
- **Echinacea**
- Licorice root
- **Ginseng**
- Zinc

Foods more widely used to relieve colds coughs, and production of mucus include:

- Lemon
- Garlic
- Spices
- Ground cayenne
- **Ginger**
- Chili pepper

Chapter 6: Dr. Sebi's Diet Plan & Recipes

This meal is designed to help you quit smoking or at least reverse the symptoms of smoking. Quitting smoking will lead to healthier pair of lungs and no mucus production.

Stop Smoking Meal Plan (3 Days)

Day 1

Breakfast: Brain-Boosting Smoothie

Lunch: Asian Cucumber Salad

Snack: Herbal tea(any)

Dinner: Mushroom Risotto

Day 2

Breakfast: Apple, pineapple & spinach smoothie

Lunch: Basil Pesto Zoodles

Snack: Herbal Tea(any)

Dinner: Cleansing Green Soup

Day 3

Breakfast: Detox Smoothie

Lunch: **Heart Friendly Salsa with Kale chips**

Snack: Herbal tea(any)

Dinner: Cauliflower Rice Bowls **Turmeric, Ginger & Kale**

By following this three-day smoke quitting meal plan. You can resist the urge to smoke that will benefit you in the long run, and your overall quality of life will improve.

Stop Smoking Diet Recipes

6.1 Blood Orange, Carrot, and Ginger Smoothie

Ingredients

- One blood orange: peeled and diced
- Almond, coconut or cashew milk: 2 cups
- Pineapple: half cup
- One knob of one inch: minced fresh ginger
- One frozen banana
- One carrot peeled and diced (medium-sized)
- Add in half apple, de-seeded and peeled
- One scoop of vegan collagen: it is optional

Instructions

- In a food blender, add all the ingredients
- Pulse on high for almost one minute, until smooth and creamy.
- Serve with fresh basil leaves on top.
- Enjoy.

6.2 Garlic and Onion Sunflower Seed Crackers

Ingredients

- Sunflower Seeds: 1 Cup
- Flax Seeds: 1/4 Cup

- Onion Powder: 1 teaspoon

- Chia Seeds: 1 teaspoon

- Nutritional Yeast Flakes: 1 teaspoon

- Himalayan Rock Salt: 1 teaspoon

- Half teaspoon of Garlic Powder

- Psyllium Husks: 1 teaspoon

- Half Cup of Water

Instructions

- Let the oven pre-heat to 360 F

- In a food blender, add the dry ingredients and pulse on high until combined and broken down, then blend more and add the water, mix well

- Prepare the baking tray with parchment paper. Lay the mixture in this baking tray and spread it.

- Spread out thinly and evenly

- Bake in the oven, for half an hour, at 360°F or until light brown

- After 20 minutes of baking, takeout from the oven and turn the tray over.

- After a total of 30 minutes, take out from the oven and let it cool.

- Break into preferred shape and size.

- For five days, you can store it in a mason jar

6.3 Garlic Miso and Onion Soup
Ingredients

- Half medium peeled yellow onion, diced

- Water: 5 cups

- Three chopped scallions

- Four cloves of pressed garlic

- Half cup of sliced shiitake mushrooms

- Garlic powder: 3/4 teaspoon

- Sesame oil: 1 teaspoon

- One silken block tofu, chopped: almost 4 cups

- Two tablespoons of soy sauce

- Miso: 1/3 cup

Instructions

- In a large pot, add all the ingredients, over medium flame, except for miso.

- Let it simmer gradually. Let it cook for 12 minutes, then add miso. Mix it well.

- Keep stirring for at least five minutes. Dissolve all the miso.

- Serve hot

6.4 Cardamom Coconut Chia Pudding

Ingredients

- Maple syrup: 2 tablespoons

- Soy or coconut milk: 2 cups

- Half cup of rolled oats (do not use instant oats)

- Three pieces of cardamom pods, crush them to expose seeds

- Ground cinnamon: 1/4 teaspoon

- Chia seeds: 4 tablespoons

Instructions

- In a jar, add all the ingredients, mix them well until well combined.

- Let it chill in Refrigerate one hour, for the very least, or up to overnight.

- Right before serving, take out the cardamom pods. Add the fruit slices (your choice).

- Add a little bit of coconut milk, if required.

- Even toddlers will enjoy this delicious recipe.

- Serve cold

6.5 Cleansing Detox Soup

Ingredients

- Vegetable broth or water: 1/4 cup

- Turmeric: 1 teaspoon

- Half of red onion, chopped

- Three stalks of chopped celery

- Three chopped medium carrots

- Two cloves of pressed garlic

- One head of small broccoli, cut into florets

- Chopped tomatoes: 1 cup

- Ginger: 1 tablespoon, peeled and freshly minced

- Cayenne pepper: 1/8 teaspoon, or to taste

- Cinnamon: 1/4 teaspoon

- Purple cabbage: 1 cup, diced

- Freshly ground black pepper, sea salt, to taste

- Water: 6 cups

- Kale: 2 cups, stem removed and torn into pieces

- Juice from half of a small lemon

Instructions

- In a big pot, over medium flame, add the vegetable broth. Once the broth is warmed, add in the garlic and onion. Cook for two minutes. Add the fresh ginger, broccoli, carrots, tomatoes, and celery.

- Cook for another three minutes. Add more water or broth if required. Add in the cayenne pepper, turmeric, cinnamon—season with pepper and salt.

- Lower the heat and let it simmer for 15 minutes. Cook until vegetables are tender.

- Add in the cabbage and kale.

- In the end, add lemon juice, let it simmer for 2-3 minutes.

- Turn off the heat

- Serve hot with fresh basil leaves.

6.6 Turmeric Smoothie

Ingredients

Turmeric Paste

- Half cup of water

- Turmeric powder: 1/4 cup

- 3/4 teaspoon of freshly ground black pepper

Smoothie

- Coconut oil: 1 teaspoon

- Prepared turmeric paste: 1 teaspoon

- Pineapple chunks: 1 cup (frozen)

- One and 1/2 cups of cold water

- Peeled ginger: 1 teaspoon (chopped fresh)

- Mango chunks: 1 cup(frozen)

Instructions

- To prepare the turmeric paste: in a pan over medium flame, mix the water with turmeric powder, until it takes the form of a paste.

- Add in the black pepper. Store the extra paste in jars for up to two weeks.

- In a food blender, add all the ingredients of smoothie.

- Pulse on high until smooth and combined

- Serve right away and enjoy.

6.7 Onion Soup with Apple

Ingredients

- Olive or coconut oil: 1 tablespoon

- Three onions (yellow & red)

- Two and a half cups of vegetable broth

- One apple

- Apple cider vinegar: 1/4 cup

- Black Pepper, to taste

- Bread(Gluten-free), for serving it is optional

Instructions

- Cut the onions into rings, after peeling them

- In a large pan, heat the oil over medium flame, cook the onions in oil for ten minutes. Do not let the onions burn.

- De-core the apples, and cut into slices. Add in the pan with onions and cook for two minutes.

- Stir in the apple cider and vegetable broth. Let it simmer for 15 to 20 minutes.

- Season with pepper or salt, if needed.

- Serve hot with fresh basil leaves on top and slices of gluten-free bread.

6.8 Arugula and Strawberry Salad with Cayenne Lemon Vinaigrette
Ingredients

Salad

- Half avocado

- Arugula: 2 cups, or greens or baby spinach (your choice)

- Walnuts (Toasted)

- Diced mango: 2 tablespoons

- Three strawberries cut into slices

- Blueberries: 1/4 cup

Dressing

- Agave syrup: 1/4 teaspoon or another sweetener

- Extra virgin olive oil: 2 tablespoons

- Powder cayenne pepper: 1/8 teaspoon

- Pinch of salt

- Lemon juice: 2 teaspoon

- Freshly ground black pepper

Instructions

- In a bowl, add all the dressing ingredients, whisk to combine, and set it aside.

- In another big bowl, add all the salad ingredients, pour the dressing all over, and top with toasted walnuts.

- Serve right away and enjoy.

6.9 Asian Cucumber Salad

Ingredients

- Grated ginger: 1 tbs.

- Key lime juice: 3 tbs.

- Half tsp. of date sugar

- powdered granulated seaweed: 1 tbs.

- Sea salt: 1/4 tsp

- Sesame oil: 1 tbs.

- Sesame seeds: 1 tbs.

Instructions

- In a big bowl, add all the ingredients. Mix them well.

- Serve with your favorite dressing.

6.10 Detox Smoothie
Ingredients

- Seville orange juice: 1 cup

- Spring water: 1 cup

- One burro banana

- Watercress: 1 cup

- One organic apple

- Blueberries: 1-2 cups

Instructions

- In a food blender, add all the ingredients,

- Pulse on high until smooth. If the smoothie is too thick, add one cup of water.

- Serve right away and enjoy.

6.11 Brain-Boosting Smoothie
Ingredients

- Half cup of raspberries

- 1 cup of Relief Herbal Tea

- Half cup blueberries

- Agave syrup: or one tablespoon of date sugar

- Half burro banana

Instructions

- In a large pan, boil one cup of water. And make the tea accordingly, letting it steep for as long as it requires, then cools it off.

- In a food blender, add the steeped tea along with all the ingredients.

- Pulse on high until well combined.

- Serve right away and enjoy.

6.12 Cleansing Green Soup

Ingredients

- Grapeseed oil: 3 tablespoons

- Three medium, two large onions: diced

- Packed dill: half cup

- Dandelion greens: one bunch

- Wild arugula: one bunch

- One zucchini, roughly diced (do not peel it)

- Packed basil: half cup

- Cayenne pepper

- One key lime: juice

- Vegetable broth: 4 cups(homemade)

- Sea salt: 1/4 teaspoon

- 1/4 of an avocado

Instructions

- In a pot, add grapeseed oil, over medium flame, until very warm.

- Add the onions, cook for five minutes, cook until translucent, then add wild arugula, dandelion green, and zucchini, cook for five minutes.

- Add the vegetable stock, let it boil, turn the heat to low, cover it, and let it simmer for at least 15 minutes.

- Now uncover it and let it cook for another 15 minutes.

- Blend with avocado, key lime juice, cayenne pepper, dill, sea salt, basil until creamy and smooth

- Season to your taste.

- Top with herbs, and serve

6.13 Heart Friendly Salsa with Kale chips

Ingredients

- Diced green bell pepper: 1/3 cup

- One cup of fresh blueberries

- One pinch of sea salt

- Grapeseed oil: 2 tbsp.

- Half diced avocado

- Two key limes (for juice only)

- Five strawberries (medium-sized)

- Red onion: 1/4

Instructions

- In a food processor, add the key lime zest and juice, strawberries, key lime juice, onion, and blueberries. Pulse until smooth.

- Season with cayenne pepper, sea salt.

- Add salsa in a bowl and mix in the chopped avocado. Enjoy with kale chips.

6.14 Basil Pesto Zoodles

Ingredients

- Cherry tomatoes: 1 cup

- Zucchini: 4 cups, cut into small strips

- One ripe avocado

- Walnuts: 1/4 cup

- Half cup packed basil leaves

- Grapeseed oil: one teaspoon

- Cayenne pepper: 1/4 teaspoon

- Extra virgin olive oil: 1/4 cup

- Sea salt: 1/2 teaspoon

Instructions

- In a pan, add grapeseed oil and sauté the zucchini noodles, until lightly tender but not mushy.

- In a food blender, add the rest of the ingredients. Pulse on high until smooth and creamy.

- If the sauce is too thick, add water.

- Coat the zoodles with sauce.

- Top with halves of cherry tomatoes and sprinkle shredded dissected coconut.
- Serve right away and enjoy.

6.15 Triple Berry Smoothie

Ingredients

- One burro banana
- Strawberries: half cup
- Agave syrup, to taste
- Blueberries: half cup
- Water: one cup
- Raspberries: half cup

Instructions

- Add all ingredients in a food blender.
- Pulse it on high until smooth and creamy. Serve and enjoy.

6.16 Apple, Pineapple Spinach Green Smoothie

Ingredients

- Baby spinach leaves: 1 cup
- Half pineapple
- Juice of one orange
- One apple
- One passion fruit (it is optional)
- Water

Garnish

- Buckwheat cereals: one teaspoon

- Chia seeds: one teaspoon

Instructions

- Cut the pineapple into chunks. Remove the core from apples, slice them. Juice the oranges after cutting into halves.

- In a food blender, add spinach leaves, orange juice, apple slices, and pineapple chunks.

- Add the passion fruit if you want. Then add water and pulse it on high. If the smoothie is very thick, adding more water if required.

- Add smoothie into glasses and serve with buckwheat cereals, chia seeds.

- Enjoy.

6.17 Mushroom Risotto

Ingredients

- Wild rice: 2 cups

- Grapeseed oil: one teaspoon

- Four mushrooms

- Half onion

- Cayenne pepper, to taste

- Homemade vegetable broth: 4 cups

- Sea salt, to taste

Instructions

- In a large pot, sauté mushrooms and onions in grapeseed oil over medium heat. Cook for 5 to 7 minutes or until mushrooms are lightly browned, and liquid is evaporated, stirring occasionally.

- Stir in rice and cook an additional minute.

- Add in the vegetable broth and additional sea salt and pepper. Cover and cook on a low-heat setting about 2 hours and 45 minutes or on a high-heat set about 1 hour 15 minutes or until rice is tender.

- Serve hot and enjoy.

6.18 Cauliflower Fried Rice with Turmeric, Ginger & Kale

Ingredients

- One large cauliflower

- Tamari soy sauce: 1 tbsp.

- Coconut oil: 1 tbsp.

- One inch of root turmeric(fresh)

- One zucchini

- Half a bunch of kale

- One inch, root ginger(fresh)

- Almonds: 2 handfuls

- One bunch of coriander

- Half a bunch of parsley

- One lime

- Spring onions: four pieces

- One bunch of mint

Instructions

- Make the cauliflower rice by chopping or grating cauliflower in a food processor.

- Thinly slice zucchini, kale, and chop (roughly) all of the herbs throw away the stems.

- Grate the turmeric and ginger after peeling them.

- Add the grated turmeric and ginger with coconut oil.

- Warm it thoroughly, add in the parsley, coriander, and mint. You can add coriander stems.

- Mix well, then add in the kale and cauliflower.

- After 2-3 minutes, add tamari, spring onions, and herbs, mix well.

- Turn off the heat. The total cooking time will be under five minutes. Do not overcook; otherwise, it will go soft.

- Stir in the roughly chop handfuls of almonds, season with pepper and salt, lime juice according to your taste.

6.19 Raw Energy Balls

Ingredients

- Brazil or walnuts nuts: half cup

- Fresh Blueberries: 1/2 cup

- Dried dates: half cup

- A pinch of sea salt

- Date sugar: one teaspoon

- Shredded soft-jelly coconut: 2 cups

- Agave syrup: 1 tablespoon

Instructions

- In a food processor, add the walnuts, pulse until finely chopped.
- Then add the blueberries, dried dates, and date sugar. Gradually add the agave syrup until fine paste forms.
- Chill in the refrigerator for half an hour to 2 hours.
- Take one tbsp. Of mixture, form into balls. Coat in dried coconut. Save in the fridge for one week or in the freezer for one month.
- Enjoy.

6.20 Green Falafels

Ingredients

- Half cup of bean flour (garbanzo)
- Beans, dry garbanzo (chickpeas): 2 cups
- Red bell pepper: 1/3 cup, diced
- Oregano: 1/4 teaspoon
- Fresh basil: 2/3 cup
- One large onion, diced
- Avocado/ Grapeseed oil for frying
- Half cup of fresh dill
- Sea salt: one teaspoon

Instructions

- Boil the chickpeas, drain the water, and wash them.

- In a food processor, add the chickpeas with the rest of the ingredients: flour, sea salt, onion, fresh herbs, red bell pepper, and oregano.

- Pulse on high until all things are finely diced and like coarse. Toss with the spoon and pulse again, taste it, and adjust the seasoning if required.

- Move this coarse meal mixture to a big mixing bowl, use your clean hands, shape them into balls or discs like structure. Place all the balls over parchment paper.

- Put in the refrigerator for one hour to chill.

- You can rather fry these falafels in one inch of oil in a deep pan. Or air fry them at 380 for ten minutes, until golden brown.

- Serve them with your favorite dipping sauce.

6.21 No Bake Energy Balls

Ingredients

- Walnuts: 1 cup

- Fresh Raspberries: 3/4 cup

- Soft-jelly coconut meat: 2 2/3 cup(shredded)

- One pinch of sea salt

- Ten dates

Instructions

- In a food processor, add all the ingredients. Pulse or mix until everything is combined.

- Use your clean, moist hands to form the energy balls. Do not need to bake them.

- After all the balls have been formed, put them in the freezer for at least half an hour.

- Serve and enjoy.

6.22 Creamy Kamut Alkaline Pasta

Ingredients

Pasta

- Box of Kamut Spirals: 1 and a half cups

- Dried tarragon: 1 tablespoon

- Spring water:6-8 cups, (to boil your pasta)

- Grapeseed oil: 2 tablespoon

- Onion powder: 1 teaspoon

- Sea salt: one teaspoon

Creamy Sauce

- Half medium onion: diced

- Grapeseed oil: divided, two tablespoon

- Sea salt + plus half teaspoon additional 1/4 teaspoon

- Spring water: 2 cups

- Freshly ground black pepper and half teaspoon more

- Sliced baby Bella mushrooms: 2 cups

- Chickpea flour: 1/4 cup

- Unsweetened can of coconut milk: one and a half cups

- Dried tarragon: 1 tablespoon

- Tomatoes(Roma), chopped 2-3

- Dried oregano: 1 teaspoon

- Onion powder: 2 teaspoon

- Fresh kale: 2 cups packed

- Dried basil: 1 teaspoon

Instructions

Pasta

- In a pot, add water with salt over high heat. Let it boil

- When the water has boiled, add pasta. Cook until tender to your preference.

- To enhance flavor, add seasoning while the pasta is still warm, add onion powder, sea salt, dried tarragon, and grapeseed oil.

- Taste the pasta and adjust the seasoning.

Creamy Sauce

- In a pan, add one tbsp. of grapeseed oil, over medium flame, heat for one minute

- In the hot oil, add in the sliced mushrooms and chopped onions. Stir often let it cook, until vegetables are tender for about five minutes.

- Add in the fresh ground black pepper and salt, 1/4 teaspoon of each. Add in chickpea flour and another one tbsp. of grapeseed oil.

- Mix constantly flour with the oil and vegetables for at least one minute. Flour should not be left dry as it will help thicken the sauce.

- Then add in the can coconut milk, dried oregano, onion powder, half a teaspoon of sea salt, dried tarragon, spring water, half a teaspoon of black pepper, and dried basil. Mix it well. Let it simmer, uncovered for 20 minutes. Or until sauce becomes thick.

- Then add in the kale, tomatoes, and seasoned, cooked pasta. Cook until the kale is wilted for five minutes. Turn off the heat.

- With time sauce will become thicker from the pasta.

- Serve with fresh basil leaves, and enjoy.

Conclusion

Dr. Sebi's Diet has immense benefits. However, it can offer some of the other advantages when linked with other diets focused on plants. Consuming more vegetables and whole fruits may have important health implications. If your target is also to also weight, it could also encourage a person to lose weight. However, the constraints of Dr. Sebi's diet may present challenges. It is important to ensure that adequate nutrients, including vitamin C, niacin amide, and vitamin B-12, are consumed by the body from supplementation if required. The risks linked with Dr. Sebi's diet could be more present in those persons. Adolescents, breastfeeding mothers, and older adults are among them because they need nutrition more than other people, and you need to take Dr. Sebi supplements if you want your body to be at its best.

Now that you have learned pretty much everything about Dr. Sebi's nutritional guide related to cleansing mucus from the body or expelling the excess of it. You want to live a healthy, balanced diet by eating more of an alkaline plant based diet. If you are a smoke or anyone around you smokes, and you get to be the target of secondhand smoke, it is in your body's best interest to take you to try to quit smoking.

Your body will thank you by showing these signs if you follow Dr. Sebi's alkaline plant-based diet to clear mucus and by stopping smoking.

- Improves digestion
- Helps in weight loss
- The healthy quality of lungs
- Reduces inflammation
- Improves liver function

- Improves skin

- Boost in immunity

- Improve Digestive Health

- Boosts energy

- Gain Control of Cravings

- Improved Emotional and Mental Health

According to a research report, the hormone cortisol is produced while we're under stress, which reduces liver function. Cleansing your body of smoking may also stabilize the amounts of cortisol, helping through the chemical change it creates to handle the tension. Processed foods, including caffeine, sugar, and alcohol, lead to adrenal exhaustion, but the adrenal glands are

strengthened through removing them from regular consumption. Good adrenal glands will assist you to interact with tension more and stop getting stressed. Also, pollutants will lead you to establish bad sleeping habits and therefore feel lethargic, which may change your mood.

Detoxifying your body through a plant-based diet would leave you feeling refreshed and rejuvenated. In the beginning, you should adapt to the elimination from your diet of some items and the results they cause. Yet you are bound to experience the beneficial effects, both emotionally and physically, until you finish the detox.

By following all these Dr. Sebi's food approved lists herbs, you can start living your new healthy life today. Cleansing your body of mucus, reversing, and unintentionally quitting smoking will do your body better than ever. You will live a healthy, sound life without any risk of major diseases.

CPSIA information can be obtained
at www.ICGtesting.com
Printed in the USA
LVHW070031271120
672786LV00027B/861